MW01148208

Fabulous Forearms
Revised Edition

Written and Published by Bill Pearl
Edited by George and Tuesday Coates
Layout and Illustrations by Richard R. Thornley Jr.

Copyright © 1963-2015 Bill Pearl

Bill Pearl
P.O. Box 1080
Phoenix, Oregon 97535
Email: support@billpearl.com
Website: www.billpearl.com

ISBN-13: 978-1-938855-07-8

Notice of Rights

Medical Disclaimer - See Your Doctor

Most people may do all of the exercises found in this book with no ill effects. However, if certain movements cause discomfort they should be eliminated. See your doctor and get the doctor's approval on the total fitness program.

Table of Contents

Chapter 1

Introduction

Forearms receive very little attention from the majority of the competitive athletes and bodybuilders. Since not enough emphasis is placed on working them, this book has been developed and published to encourage and help you to build stronger and better shaped forearms. Follow the instructions carefully and precisely. You will be amazed at how rapidly your forearms respond with this program.

Good Luck!
Leo Stern

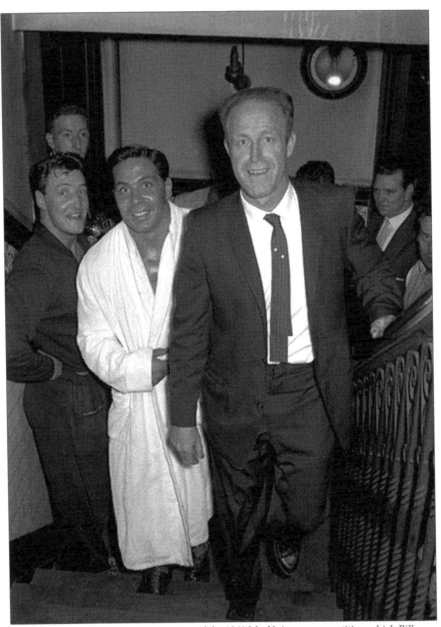

Leo Stern escorting Bill Pearl to the stage of the 1961 Mr. Universe competition which Bill won.

Chapter 2

Building Fabulous Forearms

Forearms are possibly the most overlooked muscle group of the entire physique. On rare occasions will you find a person who exercises his forearms, and then only a few of the standard movements are practiced for a short time.

Still, there are a few of our top men who seem to have "a certain something" that the others lack. If someone with an authoritative eye could point out a few details to you, the reason for this would be obvious. You would find that the champions not only have outstanding chests, shoulders, arms, legs and backs, but also the less emphasized areas, such as the calves, lower backs, trapezius, and forearms. These differences make the champions.

In my experience as a physical instructor, I have found that the athletes who come to me for professional advice have benefited nearly as much from a specialized program for their forearms as they have from any specialized training. If you stop to analyze how much you use your forearms in all major sports, such as football, track, field events, wrestling, and baseball, you can realize why it is so important to develop and strengthen these muscles. For example, I have seen world champion track men set new records in the shot putt and discus, simply by adding forearm exercises to their training programs. I have seen a world's champion water skier set new world records in speed racing simply because he started working on his grip and strengthened his forearms. This enabled him to take the strain of being pulled at nearly 115 miles per hour behind a boat. I can name several other instances such as these.

You may not be interested in setting world records in track or water skiing, but if you were able to eliminate an injury to the wrists and elbows during your particular sports season, it would be worth the effort to work and condition these forearm muscles.

You may not be interested in entering physique contests, still, no harm can be done in having a set of forearms that will reveal you as a person who takes considerable pride in himself. People may not be able to see how big your deltoids are or how large your upper arm is under a short sleeved shirt, but they can see your forearms. A set of well-developed forearms has been a sign of power and strength since the beginning of time.

Add this training to your program and stick with it. As your forearms continue to improve, you will become more and more enthused about working them. Eventually, you will not think of leaving these exercises out of your training program. You will be surprised at the many favorable comments your large, well-shaped, muscular forearms will bring.

Best of Luck,
Bill Pearl

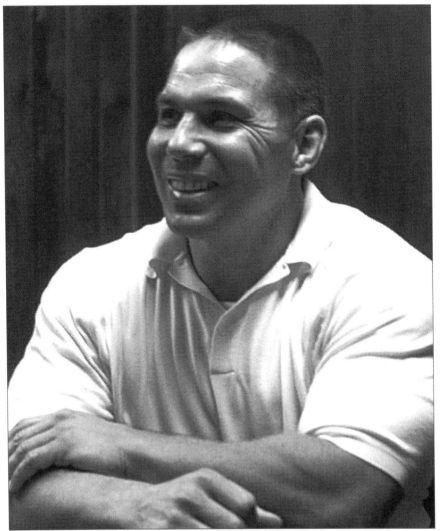

Bill Pearl smiling after a good days work.

Chapter 3

How to Use this Book

If a person is interested in weight training for more than basic conditioning, it is imperative that they study each illustration and description before attempting a new exercise. Progress definitely can be deterred if an exercise is done incorrectly.

Many exercises can be accomplished with the exact same motion but will affect different areas of a muscle by the angle at which the exercise is performed. For example: an exercise done on a flat bench, or an incline bench, will put different emphasis on the same muscle even though the same motion, weight and equipment are used.

It is therefore necessary to perform exercises from as many different angles that are reasonable and to use as many variations that are reasonable to develop a fully matured muscular physique.

On the following pages, highly accurate drawings appear that will enable you to see the pieces of equipment used to perform each exercise and the style used for each movement. Each exercise includes the proper name of the exercise, the muscle group most affected, "degree of difficulty" information, and a written description of how the exercise should be done.

The "degree of difficulty" information appearing below each exercise heading will give you at a glance what exercise may be suited for your present physical condition.

NOTE: It is not necessarily true that an exercise considered "easy" may not be just as effective as one considered "hard". Any exercise can be made more or less difficult, depending on the weight used or the effort put forth.

This booklet contains basic, proven facts on developing powerful, well-shaped forearms. Although no set rule can be applied to each individual, there are certain basic principles that can be followed by everyone.

Listed in this booklet are six excellent exercises for the extensor muscles of the outer forearm and six exercises for the flexor muscles of the inner forearm. Because all of the exercises involve a complete contraction and extension of the forearm, they are equally beneficial.

Any movement that involves a fairly complete contraction and extension of the wrist and has a resistance factor included, will cause a beneficial effect

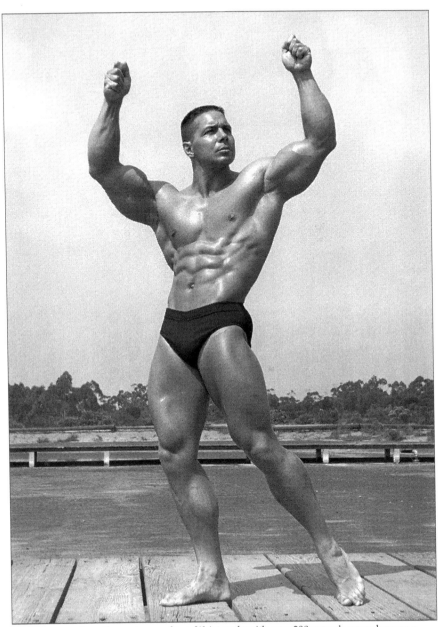

Bill's forearm strength was tremendous. Wrist curls with over 200 pounds were done on a regular daily basis. He always worked his forearms hard.

on the forearms as far as strength, size and shape is concerned. Because of this, most body builders, weight lifters, gymnasts and wrestlers should have a better than average forearm. In nearly every case, it has been proven that with a specialization program on the forearms, the effect on the individual has been well worth the effort. It is extremely important that you start with a light weight if you have not been specializing on your forearms. Too much strain on the wrist, caused from the stretching, can cause considerable pain that may last for weeks. You will also notice that you will not be able to handle nearly as much weight in any of the outer forearm exercises as you can for the inner forearm work. This is because of the difference in the size and strength of the two muscle groups.

In beginning your specialization program, which should be done approximately three times a week, choose one exercise for the inner and one for the outer forearm. Begin with your exercise for the inner forearm and perform the exercise for three sets of 10 repetitions. After a brief rest, commence with the exercise you have chosen for the outer forearm and perform three sets of 10 reps. Add a set for each muscle group every week until you have six sets for each muscle group. If the weights become light as you progress, add a few pounds from time to time, until it becomes an effort to do the last few repetitions of each set. After you have gone through this breaking-in period, which should take about 6 weeks, choose two different exercises from the lists.

After the beginning program has been completed, there are two separate advanced programs. One is devoted to power and the other to muscularity. Either or both of these programs may be used.

The power program starts with a weight you can handle for five sets of 15 reps. Each week try to add five pounds to the exercises and keep the reps at 15. If you stay on this method of training for any length of time, you will be amazed at your strength. The longer you stay on this type of program the more power you will develop. Eventually you will be using weights that were impossible for you to handle a few months earlier.

The muscularity program uses more reps rather than added weight. It also may be used to give variety to the power program. Start with six sets of 20 reps and add 5 reps each week. In one month, you will be up to 40 reps per set and your forearms will take on a hard muscular look that will give you more stamina and gripping power in the lower arms.

If your forearms are small and obtaining size is important to you, spend more time on the inner forearm after you have finished your initial training period. Until you have obtained the girth you feel is right for you, pick two exercises for the inner forearm and perform four sets for each exercise for a total of eight sets. You can experiment on the weight and reps as you go along for the sake of deviation.

By alternating the different exercises month to month, you will find you can obtain different combinations and this will give you enough of a varied program to keep the exercises interesting to you. With a little experimenting on your part, you will notice after a few months that a certain amount of sets and reps seem to have a better effect on your forearms. This is the key you should be looking for and eventually should use most of the time. It is still advisable to change the exercises as you go along because it will work the muscle groups at different angles and give you a better overall development.

Chapter 4

Do's and Don'ts

- Do a complete extension and contraction.
- Do all the seated exercises on a bench no higher than 18 inches.
- Do your forearm work after all your upper body exercises are completed.
- Do all movements with poundage that will allow you to complete the recommended sets and repetitions.
- Do all the exercises at a reasonable speed to keep the muscles warm.
- Don't cheat on any of the exercises.
- Don't allow the weight to roll down the fingers - keep the hands closed with a good grip on the bar at all times.
- Study the illustrations and instructions. They are your guide to doing the exercises correctly.

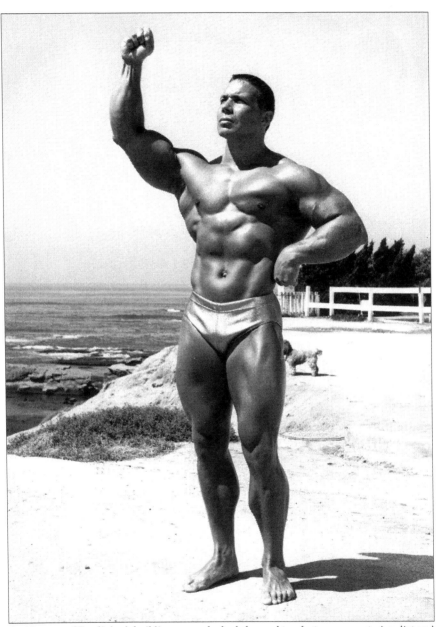

At this stage of Pearl's bodybuilding career, he had changed to a lacto-ovo-vegetarian diet and was still able to maintain his massive size. His forearms, in particular, standout in this photo by Leo Stern.

Chapter 5

Equipment Needed

Equipment needed to perform the exercises in this training guide.

- Barbell
- Dumbbells
- Flat Bench
- Ball
- Hand Gripper
- Newspaper

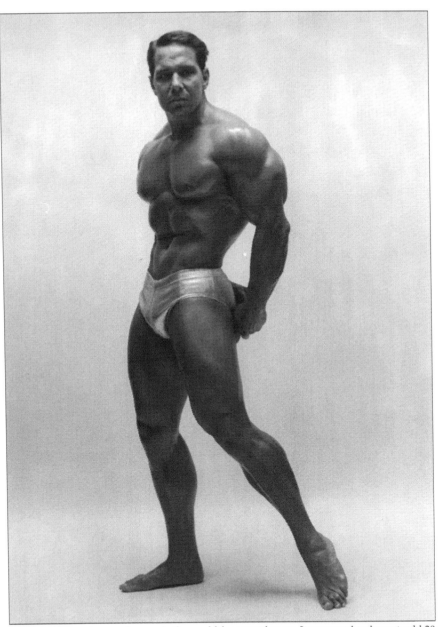

Bill had the largest muscular arm in the world for several years. It measured an honest cold 20 3/8 inches at a body weigh of 218.

Chapter 6

Flexor Exercises

SQUATTING BARBELL PALMS UP WRIST CURL

Muscle Group: Inside forearms
Degree of Difficulty: Intermediate

Grasp a barbell with both hands using a palms up grip about sixteen inches wide. Squat down until your upper thighs are parallel with the floor. Lean forward and place your forearms on your upper thighs, keeping your palms facing down. Have your hands over your knees at your wrists. Lower the bar to the lowest possible comfortable position by bending your wrists downward but keeping a tight grip on the bar throughout the exercise. Inhale and curl your hands upward as high as you possibly can. Do not let your forearms raise up from your upper thighs. Lower the weight to starting position and exhale.

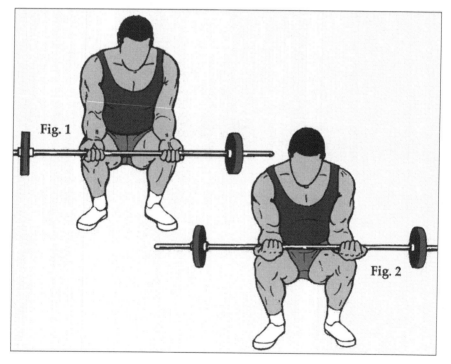

Fig. 1

Fig. 2

SEATED BARBELL PALMS UP WRIST CURL

Muscle Group: Inside forearms
Degree of Difficulty: Intermediate
Grasp a barbell with both hands using a palms up grip about sixteen inches wide. Sit at the end of a bench and plant your feet on the floor about twelve inches apart. Lean forward and place your forearms on your upper thighs, keeping your palms facing up. Have your hands over your knees just at your wrists. Lower the bar to the lowest possible comfortable position by bending your wrists downward but keep a tight grip on the bar throughout the exercise. Inhale and curl your hands upward as high as you possibly can. Do not let your forearms raise up from your upper thighs. Lower the weight to starting position and exhale.

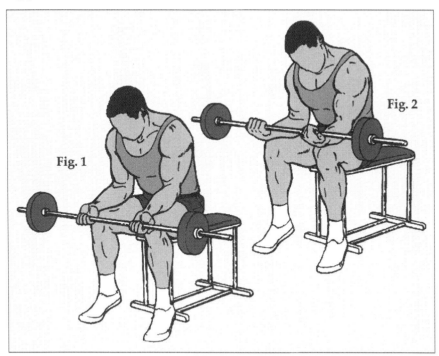

Fig. 1

Fig. 2

BARBELL OVER A BENCH PALMS UP WRIST CURL

Muscle Group: Inside forearms
Degree of Difficulty: Intermediate

Place a barbell beside a flat bench that is about sixteen inches high. Kneel down on your knees on the opposite side of the bench. Reach over and grasp the barbell with both hands, using a palms up grip about sixteen inches wide. Pick the bar up and place your forearms flat on the bench. Have your hands over the side of the bench just at your wrists. Lower the barbell to the lowest possible comfortable position by bending your wrist downward, but keep a tight grip on the bar throughout the exercise. Inhale and curl your hands upward as high as you possibly can. Do not let your forearms raise up from the bench. Lower the weight to starting position and exhale.

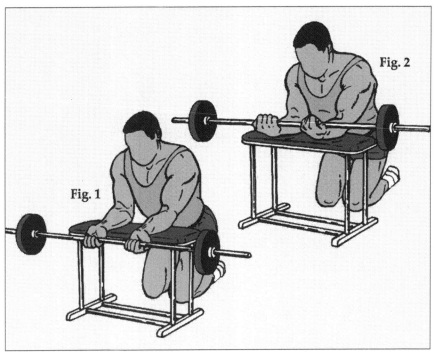

Fig. 2

Fig. 1

SEATED TWO DUMBBELL PALMS UP WRIST CURL

Muscle Group: Inside forearms
Degree of Difficulty: Intermediate

Grasp a dumbbell in each hand. Sit at the end of a flat bench and plant your feet on the floor about twelve inches apart. Lean forward and place your forearms on your upper thighs keeping your palms facing up. Have your hands over your knees just at your wrists. Lower the dumbbells to the lowest possible comfortable position by bending your wrists downward but keep a tight grip on the dumbbells throughout the exercise. Inhale and curl your hands upward as high as you possibly can. Do not let your forearms raise up from your upper thighs. Lower the weights to starting position and exhale.

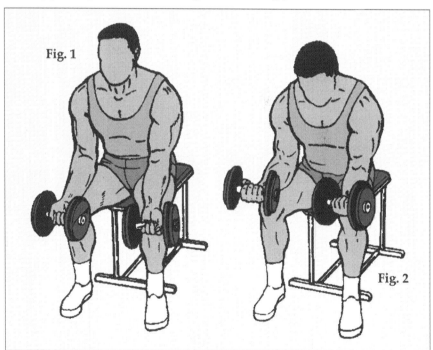

Fig. 1

Fig. 2

TWO DUMBBELL OVER A BENCH PALMS UP WRIST CURL

Muscle Group: Inside forearms
Degree of Difficulty: Intermediate

Place two dumbbells beside a flat bench that is about sixteen inches high. Kneel down on your knees on the opposite side of the bench. Reach over and grasp the dumbbells with both hands. Pick the dumbbells up and place your forearms flat on the bench. Have your hands over the side of the bench just at your wrist with your palms up and about sixteen inches apart. Lower the dumbbells to the lowest possible comfortable position by bending your wrists downward, but keep a tight grip on the weights throughout the exercise. Inhale and curl your hands upward as high as you possibly can. Do not let your forearms raise up from the bench. Lower the weights to starting position and exhale.

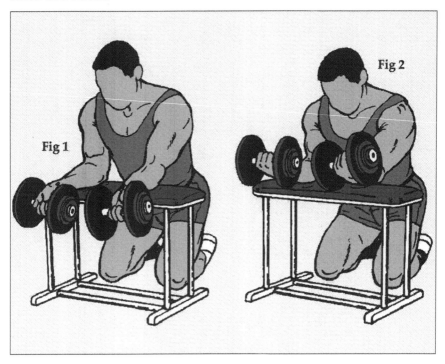

STANDING BEHIND BACK BARBELL PALMS UP WRIST CURL

Muscle Group: Inside forearms
Degree of Difficulty: Intermediate

Place a barbell on the floor. Step over the bar and squat down and pick the bar up, using a palms away grip about twenty inches wide as you stand erect and place the bar where your buttocks and upper thighs meet. Keep your back and arms straight with your elbows locked. Inhale and curl your hands upward as high as you possibly can. Lower the bar to starting position and exhale.

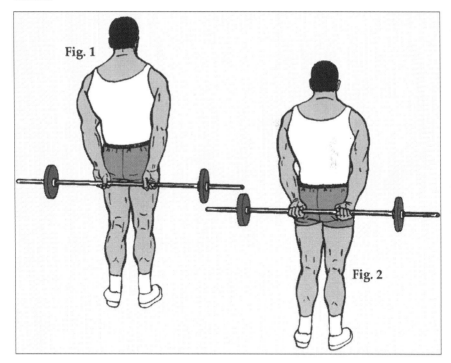

Fig. 1

Fig. 2

Chapter 7

Extensor Exercises

SQUATTING BARBELL PALMS DOWN WRIST CURL

Muscle Group: Outside forearms
Degree of Difficulty: Intermediate

Grasp a barbell with both hands, using a palms down grip about ten inches wide. Squat down until your upper thighs are parallel with the floor. Lean forward and place your forearms on your upper thighs keeping your palms facing down. Have your hands over your knees at your wrists. Lower the bar to the lowest possible comfortable position by bending your wrists downward but keeping a tight grip on the bar throughout the exercise. Inhale and curl your hands upward as high as you possibly can. Do not let your forearms raise up from your upper thighs. Lower the weight to starting position and exhale.

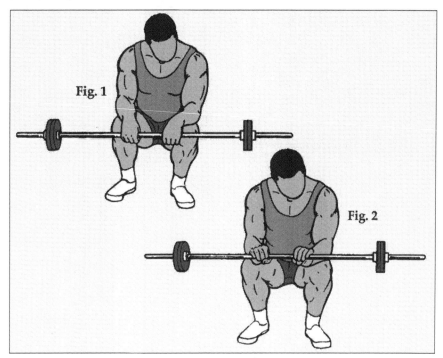

Fig. 1

Fig. 2

SEATED BARBELL PALMS DOWN WRIST CURL

Muscle Group: Outside forearms
Degree of Difficulty: Intermediate

Grasp a barbell with both hands using a palms down grip about ten inches wide. Sit at the end of a bench and plant your feet on the floor about twelve inches apart. Lean forward and place your forearms on your upper thighs, keeping your palms facing down. Have your hands over your knees just at your wrists. Lower the bar to the lowest possible comfortable position by bending your wrists downward but keeping a tight grip on the bar throughout the exercise. Inhale and curl your hands upward as high as you possibly can. Do not let your forearms raise up from your upper thighs. Lower the weight to starting position and exhale.

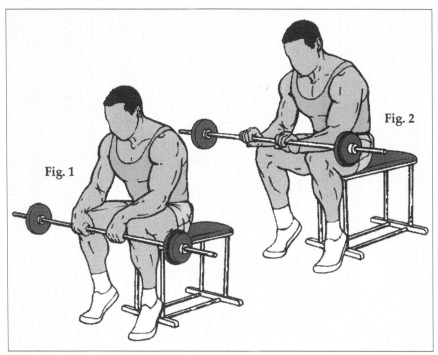

Fig. 1

Fig. 2

BARBELL OVER A BENCH PALMS DOWN WRIST CURL

Muscle Group: Outside forearms
Degree of Difficulty: Intermediate

Place a barbell beside a flat bench that is about sixteen inches high. Kneel down on your knees on the opposite side of the bench. Reach over and grasp the barbell with both hands, using a palms down grip about twelve inches wide. Pick the bar up and place your forearms flat on the bench. Have your hands over the side of the bench just at your wrists. Lower the barbell to the lowest possible comfortable position by bending your wrists downward but keep a tight grip on the bar throughout the exercise. Inhale and curl your hands upward as high as you possibly can. Do not let your forearms raise up from the bench. Lower the weight to starting position and exhale.

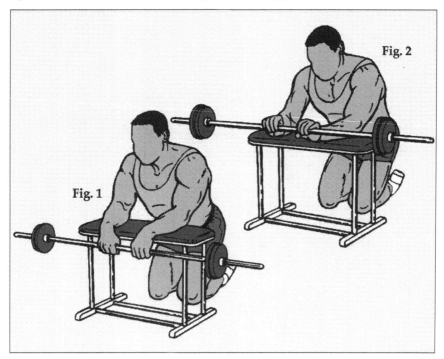

Fig. 1

Fig. 2

SEATED BARBELL PALMS DOWN WRIST CURL

Muscle Group: Outside forearms
Degree of Difficulty: Intermediate

Grasp a barbell with both hands using a palms down grip about ten inches wide. Sit at the end of a bench and plant your feet on the floor about twelve inches apart. Lean forward and place your forearms on your upper thighs, keeping your palms facing down. Have your hands over your knees just at your wrists. Lower the bar to the lowest possible comfortable position by bending your wrists downward but keeping a tight grip on the bar throughout the exercise. Inhale and curl your hands upward as high as you possibly can. Do not let your forearms raise up from your upper thighs. Lower the weight to starting position and exhale

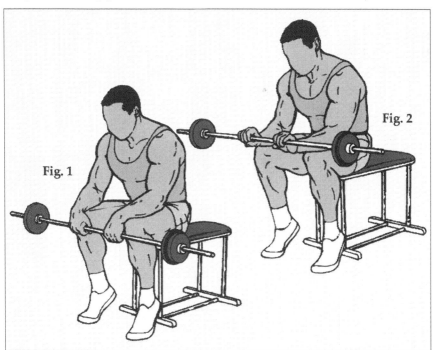

Fig. 1

Fig. 2

SEATED TWO DUMBBELL PALMS DOWN WRIST CURL

Muscle Group: Outside forearms
Degree of Difficulty: Intermediate

Grasp a dumbbell in each hand. Sit at the end of a flat bench and plant your feet on the floor about twelve inches apart. Lean forward and place your fore-arms on your upper thighs, keeping your palms facing down. Have your hands over your knees just at your wrists. Lower the dumbbells to the lowest possible comfortable position by bending your wrists downward, but keep a tight grip on the dumbbells throughout the exercise. Inhale and curl your hands upward as high as possible. Do not let your forearms raise up from your upper thighs. Lower the weights to starting position and exhale.

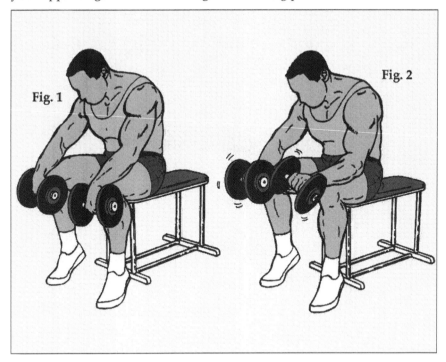

Fig. 1

Fig. 2

TWO DUMBBELL OVER A BENCH PALMS DOWN WRIST CURL

Muscle Group: Outside forearms
Degree of Difficulty: Intermediate

Place two dumbbells beside a flat bench that is about sixteen inches high. Kneel down on your knees on the opposite side of the bench. Reach over and grasp the dumbbells with both hands. Pick the dumbbells up and place your forearms flat on the bench. Have your hands over the side of the bench just at your wrists with your palms down and about twelve inches apart. Lower the dumbbells to the lowest possible comfortable position by bending your wrists downward but keep a tight grip on the weights throughout the exercise. Inhale and curl your hands upward as high as you possibly can. Do not let your forearms raise up from the bench. Lower the weights to starting position and exhale.

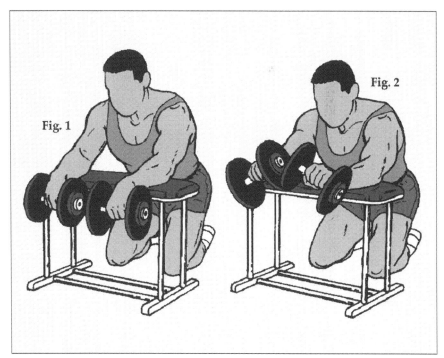

Fig. 1   Fig. 2

Grip and Forearm Exercises

NEWSPAPER HAND AND FOREARM EXERCISE

Muscle Group: Hand and forearm muscles
Degree of Difficulty: Intermediate

This exercise can be done numerous ways. It can be done standing, seated, lying, etc. The only thing required to perform the exercise is a fairly large piece of paper such as a sheet of newspaper. The object of the exercise is to start at one corner of the paper and commence to gather it into the palm of your hand. Continue gathering the paper and compress it into a small, compact unit in the palm of your hand.

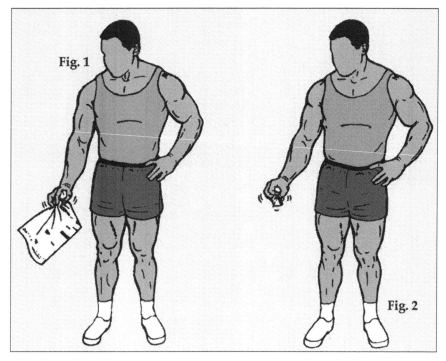

NEWSPAPER HAND AND FOREARM EXERCISE

Muscle Group: Hand and forearm muscles
Degree of Difficulty: Intermediate

This exercise can be done numerous ways. It can be done standing, seated, lying, etc. The only thing required to perform the exercise is a fairly large piece of paper such as a sheet of newspaper. The object of the exercise is to start at one corner of the paper and commence to gather it into the palm of your hand. Continue gathering the paper and compress it into a small, compact unit in the palm of your hand.

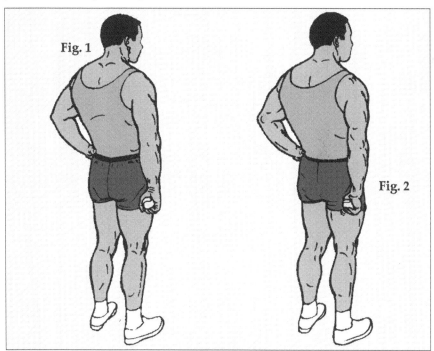

Fig. 1

Fig. 2

HAND GRIPPER FOREARM EXERCISER

Muscle Group: Hand and forearm muscles
Degree of Difficulty: Intermediate

This exercise can be done numerous ways. It can be done standing, seated, etc. The object of the exercise is to grasp the handles as tightly as you can. Some grippers are designed so they are unable to completely touch the handles together while others are not set up as tight. Continue squeezing the handles together until your grip or forearms start to give out and then change to the other hand, repeating the exercise.

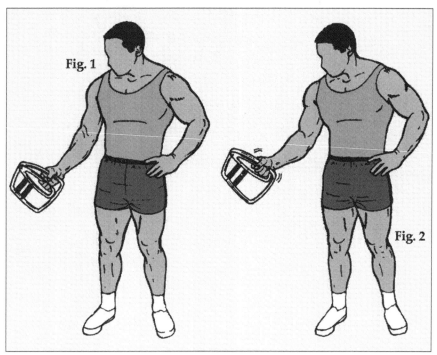

Made in the USA
San Bernardino, CA
27 July 2018